D1825642

Managing ADHD

Take Control of ADHD Naturally with Diet and Supplements

Christine Weil

Christine Weil

© 2014

All Rights Reserved. No part of this publication may be reproduced in any form or by any means, including scanning, photocopying, or otherwise without prior written permission of the copyright holder.

Disclaimer and Terms of Use: The Author and Publisher have strived to be as accurate and complete as possible in the creation of this book, notwithstanding the fact that they do not warrant or represent at any time that the contents within are accurate due to the rapidly changing nature of the Internet. While all attempts have been made to verify information provided in this publication, the Author and Publisher assume no responsibility for errors, omissions, or contrary interpretation of the subject matter herein. Any perceived slights of specific persons, peoples, or organizations are unintentional. In practical advice books, like anything else in life, there are no guarantees of income made or health benefits received. This book is not intended for use as a source of medical, legal, business, accounting or financial advice. All readers are advised to seek services of competent professionals in medical, legal, business, accounting, and finance matters.

Printed in the United States of America

Table of Contents

Introduction

I want to thank you and congratulate you for purchasing, *"Natural Health & Natural Cures Series – Naturally Treating Your ADHD."*

This book contains valuable information on natural and holistic approaches to managing ADHD and its symptoms.

If you are reading this guide, then chances are you or someone you know is looking for natural options for treating ADHD. The information provided in this guide provides an outline of the most effective and commonly used natural treatment options, information on what symptoms each option can be used to address, and action you can take to incorporate that treatment option into an overall ADHD management program.

Thank you again for purchasing this book; I hope you enjoy it!

Christine Weil

Treating ADHD 101

Despite being one of the most talked about mental health conditions, most people know very little about ADHD. This is due in part to many misconceptions about the disorder. One of the most common misconceptions is that it isn't real, that it was made up by the pharmaceutical industry in order to sell stimulant medication.

The truth is, the symptoms that are now grouped together and called ADHD have been documented for more than 100 years. We also know, based on research conducted over the last decade, that ADHD is a brain-based disorder, and that those with the condition display differences in brain structure and neurotransmitter ratio when compared to the brains of those without the condition.

The other most common misconception is that the only way to treat ADHD is with stimulant medication. The truth is that medication can be very effective at alleviating the symptoms many people with ADHD experience but medication doesn't work for about 1 in 5 people with ADHD. Additionally, the side effects that can be experienced with ADHD medications can cause severe enough side effects in some people that they cannot use medication as part of their treatment and management program.

Thankfully, there are many natural and holistic ways to make ADHD and its specific symptoms easier to manage. In fact, it is generally recommended that even those who take medication also use other supportive therapies and natural remedies in addition to their medication in order to get the best possible result.

The remaining chapters of this guide will explore the various natural and holistic options that can be beneficial in managing

ADHD. Not all natural remedies will work for everyone with ADHD because ADHD is such an individual condition. Some of the natural cures work best for specific symptoms. Just as with medication, which often requires several adjustments in order to find the right medication at the right dose, it may take some trial and error to determine which natural remedies and holistic treatments provide the most benefit.

ADHD Coaching

After medication, ADHD coaching is the most effective treatment option for everyone impacted by ADHD. ADHD coaches are specially trained life coaches who work with individuals with ADHD and their families to find the right strategies, techniques, and tactics to tackle the ADHD symptoms that are causing impairment.

One of the reasons coaching is so beneficial is that each program can be tailored to meet the individual needs of a specific client. This means that the actual symptoms and issues a person, family, or couple is dealing with can be addressed. Coaches focus on empowering those with ADHD to take action and develop the skills and strategies they need to self-manage their symptoms. The supportive environment allows those with the disorder to try different approaches to managing symptoms and overcoming challenges.

Coaches can also help individuals and those who support them to learn about their individual ADHD and how it affects their lives. Using their special training, in-depth knowledge of ADHD, and experience coaching others with similar problems, ADHD coaches help those with ADHD build a lifestyle and environment that is supportive, structured, and ADHD-friendly.

When choosing a coach to work with, people should look for coaches who have received training as a life coach, plus specific training in how to coach those with ADHD. Many coaches specialize in working with a particular type of client like teenagers or college students. Working with a coach whose experience is specific to an individual's circumstances or life stage can be very beneficial.

When looking for an ADHD coach, individuals and families should consider the following:

1. Training

Because life coaching in general and ADHD coaching specifically are not generally regulated like other mental health or medical professions, those seeking the services of an ADHD coach need to do their homework. Choosing a coach that is a certified ADHD coach ensures they have been trained to provide the services being requested. Certification can be done through the International Coaching Federation, ADDCA (The ADD Coaching Academy) and the Professional Association of ADHD Coaches.

2. Experience with ADHD

In addition to training and certification, choose a coach that has experience with ADHD. As coaching is a relatively new profession, finding a local coach with years of experience providing ADHD coaching services may be difficult. However, experience with ADHD as a parent, sibling, spouse, or even as someone who also has the disorder can give a newer coach the insight and experience they need to make a difference in the lives of those with the disorder.

3. Fit

The relationship between a coach and a client works best when they have a connection and feel comfortable with each other. Finding a coach who is a good fit will increase the likelihood that the coaching process will be successful. Working with a coach whose specialty meets the specific needs of a client is one example of finding a coach that fits. Fit is about more than just matching specialty to need. It is about getting a good vibe, feeling comfortable, and establishing a quick and easy connection.

4. Professional Demeanor

Expectations for working with an ADHD coach should be the same as they would be if you were working with a therapist, medical doctor, or other health professional. All coaches should provide upfront pricing information and an explanation of their policies and procedures, especially those related to missed appointments, package pricing, refunds, privacy, and confidentiality.

Working with an ADHD coach can help those with ADHD and their families and spouses understand the disorder, build skills to overcome the challenges it can create, and build a safety net that is empowering. ADHD coaching is very beneficial for those who choose not to take medication as well as for those that do.

Stress Management

It seems like everyone in today's society is suffering from excessive stress, and those with ADHD are no exception. In addition to dealing with the normal everyday stress that everyone experiences, those with ADHD also have to deal with the stress that comes from struggling to do common, everyday things that are easy for those without the disorder. Unfortunately, this extra stress is even more detrimental than it might be in someone without ADHD. This is because stress exacerbates ADHD symptoms, making them worse.

This is true for all kinds of stress, including the stress described above, as well as anything that is stressful to the body like bad habits and food sensitivities. This means that when we talk about using stress management as a natural way to manage ADHD, we are talking about adopting the kind of healthy lifestyle that addresses the physical needs, as well as using traditional stress management techniques to manage and decrease the amount of everyday stress the person with ADHD is under.

The importance of using healthy lifestyle habits like getting adequate sleep, eating right, acknowledging and avoiding food sensitivities, and getting enough exercise as a natural strategy for managing ADHD will be covered in subsequent chapters. The following are natural and holistic ways to manage the other kinds of stress in order to decrease the impact of stress on ADHD symptoms.

Traditional Relaxation Techniques

Relaxation techniques like meditation, guided meditation, deep breathing, massage, interacting with nature, and yoga can all be used to help keep stress levels in check.

Meditation

Traditional meditation, which most people believe requires you to sit still and quiet for long periods of time, may seem like a bad fit for people with ADHD. It can actually be very beneficial. Meditation helps people with ADHD get off the adrenaline roller-coaster many use to help them cope with their condition. Whether consciously or subconsciously, it is common for people with ADHD to realize that, even with their ADHD brain, crisis always equates to action. This can create an unhealthy dynamic where everything gets turned into a crisis and even everyday life events become filled with drama. In essence, these people become addicted to being stressed out.

As outlined above, stress and ADHD are a bad combination, and meditation can help those with ADHD step off of the adrenaline rollercoaster. Research has shown that practicing mindfulness meditation reduces a person's level of cortisol, the hormone released in the body in response to stress. It is even being used in the U.S. military as a way to help soldiers manage the stress of being on the battlefield. Meditation is such a powerful tool for managing stress that it is also used to decrease stress among those undergoing treatment for cancer.

Meditation can also be beneficial at alleviating and/or managing ADHD symptoms. One study showed that people who meditated were able to improve their working memory abilities. The authors of that study believe meditation may actually have more wide-spread effect on cognitive functioning as well. Other research indicates that meditative practices help people learn to control their focus and better regulate their emotions, both of which are beneficial to those with ADHD. Meditation can also help lower the risk of depression which is commonly co-morbid with ADHD.

Fortunately, contrary to popular opinion, you do not have to sit still and quiet or be able to clear your mind in order to meditate. In fact, there are several accepted meditation practices, like walking in nature and chanting, that can be perfectly suited to people with ADHD. The key to success is to create a meditation practice that suits the individual.

Guided Meditation

Guided meditation is another way that people with ADHD can get some of the benefits of meditation. Where mindfulness meditation is inwardly directed, guided meditation is directed by an external entity. In guided mediation, an individual is guided by another, usually a voice recording, through a series of instructions that clear the mind and relax the body. During guided meditation, individuals focus their attention, engage their imagination, and pay attention to their breathing.

Guided meditation can be very powerful in helping people create change in their lives, which is one of the other ways it can benefit those with ADHD. When the imagination is engaged, the brain can create powerful visualizations. The brain doesn't differentiate between these imagined things and those things that are real. This makes it possible for individuals with ADHD to use specific visualization exercises as part of guided meditation in order to change habits and make other positive lifestyle changes.

Choosing guided meditation experiences that align with the personal change goals that need to be achieved can help those with ADHD as they learn new ways to manage their symptoms. It can be very supportive in helping to anchor a new way of thinking or a new habit.

Deep Breathing Exercises

Deep breathing exercises can provide stress management benefits to anyone, including people with ADHD. One of the most powerful and immediate benefits those with ADHD can experience when they breathe deeply is that is slows things down. It slows the pulse, lowers the heart rate, and can help slow down emotions and thoughts as well. The ability to slow things down, even for only a few seconds, can make a significant difference for those who struggle with emotional disregulation, impulsive behavior, and angry outbursts.

Deep breathing has many health benefits but for those with ADHD. It can be used to mitigate some of the most challenging symptoms stemming from impulsivity. Taking a deep breath can make it easier not to interrupt other people while they are talking. Deep breathing can make it easier to wait in lines or sit in traffic and help keep the frustration and anger that many with ADHD experience in these situations from taking hold.

Deep breathing is also a powerful stress reliever that can be used anywhere. Simply taking a few deep breaths reduces tension, loosens muscles, and makes it easier to reign in and control powerful emotions.

For those who struggle with mental hyperactivity, deep breathing can help wrangle all those rapid-fire thoughts into a calmer stream of consciousness. It can help focus attention, and in many cases simply breathing deeply can be a powerful tool that allows those with ADHD to continue paying attention in circumstances where that can be difficult. For example, an adult who struggles to sustain their attention during long meetings can use deep breathing techniques to keep their attention from wavering.

There are a wide variety of deep breathing techniques available that can easily be learned and incorporated into everyday life. For many with ADHD, simply learning the proper way to breathe can make a significant difference in their ability to manage the normal stresses and frustrations that occur each day. Adding a few easy and unobtrusive deep breathing techniques to that knowledge provides a quick and always available way to calm their emotions, refocus their minds, and take the second or two they need to employ a symptom-management strategy or tactic.

Most people today do not breathe properly; they breathe shallowly through their mouth into their chest. Proper breathing flows through nose into the abdomen, engaging the diaphragm before filling the lungs and chest. Deep breathing is slow and rhythmic. Here is a very basic deep breathing exercise that those with ADHD can use to slow things down.

1. Breathe in through the nose to a count of 4 or 5.
2. Pull the air all the way into the abdomen, letting the belly expand before the lungs.
3. Expand the lungs and chest.
4. Hold for a count of 3.
5. Release the air slowly through the mouth to a count of 4 or 5.

For the best benefit, this exercise should be done for 10 minutes at a time, two times each day. It can also be done as needed for immediate stress relief or to help manage emotions.

Massage

Getting a massage can be deeply relaxing, but for people with ADHD, massage offers benefits that go beyond the time spent on the massage bed. Research indicates that adolescents who regularly received biweekly massages saw improvements in their overall mood and behavior after only a few weeks. Other research indicates that regular massages may also help to alleviate hyperactivity and the constant restlessness many people with ADHD experience.

Interacting with Nature

One of the most powerful stress-management tools every person with ADHD has is right outside their door – nature. Often referred to as "green time," spending time outdoors in open green spaces has been proven to have a positive effect on children and adults with ADHD. Past research has shown that simply stepping outside into a open green space for a few minutes offers a short-term boost in impulse control and concentration for those with ADHD. Further research indicates that when "green-time" is part of a regular ADHD management program it helps improve behavior across the board.

Initial theories attribute the "green-time" effect to a boost in brain stimulation that helps increase and focus attention in the time immediately following the exposure. Research has shown that when any brain, ADHD or not, is required to sustain focus and attention on something for too long, it becomes fatigued. Exposing that brain to a natural setting, like a park, a lightly wooded trail, a flower garden, or some other green space, can fight that fatigue and boost the brain's ability to remain focused. In one study, people improved their scores on tests of memory and attention after taking a short walk through a tree-filled park.

When seeking green-time as part of an ADHD management program, it is important to note that simply going outside will not produce the expected benefit. Green-time is time spent in an open space with lots of green present and city streets lined with skyscrapers or suburban streets full of cars and houses are not going to produce the same effect. The soccer field at a school, the botanical garden in a city, or a large park can all be good spaces for getting in some green-time.

While there is no clear recommendation on the ratio amount of green time to length of short-term benefits, research shows benefits after as little as 20 minutes spent outside. In order to achieve a longer term benefit to behavior, those with ADHD should dedicate a certain amount of time each day to being in open green spaces.

Yoga

Yoga is widely accepted as being beneficial for stress management. It is covered in more depth within the "Exercise" chapter of this guide.

Sleep

One of the challenges many people with ADHD experience is sleep disturbances, although there isn't a clear indication as to why. For some, falling asleep is a challenge because of mental or physical hyperactivity. For others, their body clock seems to want to follow a different sleep/wake cycle than the one society dictates. Regardless of why those with ADHD have so much trouble sleeping, sleep deprivation has a negative impact on most ADHD symptoms. Just like stress, lack of sleep makes ADHD worse.

Research has shown that getting the right amount of sleep on a regular basis is critical for every aspect of our health. Sleep deprivation impacts everything from our metabolism to our life expectancy. One of the first things lack of sleep impacts is our cognitive abilities. Unfortunately for those with ADHD, these are the same functions that many already struggle with, which means that not getting enough sleep only makes things that are already challenging even harder to overcome.

There are some sleep disorders that commonly occur with ADHD like insomnia and sleep apnea. For this reason, it is important to work with a medical professional to rule out any underlying sleep disorders as the first step.

Additionally, people with ADHD can benefit greatly from practicing good sleep hygiene which includes:

- Going to bed and getting up at the same time every day, even on weekends
- Establishing a regular bedtime routine that uses relaxation techniques to help the body get ready for sleep.
- Eating right.

- Getting exercise every day, early in the day.
- Avoiding caffeine and naps after 3 PM.
- Eating no food less than two hours before bedtime.
- Controlling the sleep environment to eliminate any light or sound that can disrupt sleep.
- Avoiding any stimulating activities in the hours before sleep.
- Avoiding electronic screens like televisions, computers, and cell phones in the hour or two before bed.
- Creating a comfortable sleep environment that is inviting and promotes sleep.
- Using the bedroom only for sleeping and sex.

Some people with ADHD struggle with sleep because they cannot get their mind to "shut down." For these people, taking a few minutes to record those racing thoughts on paper may help alleviate this problem.

Others struggle to stop doing something they enjoy so that they can go to sleep on time. This can be one of the most difficult ADHD sleep challenges to overcome, and why it is so important to avoid stimulating activities and follow a set routine when it is time to go to sleep.

Hyperactivity can also cause sleep problems for some people with ADHD. The best way to burn off excess hyperactive energy is usually to do something physical, but exercise that elevates your body temperature in the hours before bedtime can keep you from sleeping. For those whose hyperactivity keeps them from sleeping, light yoga, deep breathing, and other relaxation techniques can help release some of the hyperactive energy without impeding your sleep.

Additionally, some people who take medication for their ADHD have trouble sleeping because of the medication.

Those who take ADHD medication and experience difficulties with sleep should work with their prescribing doctor to determine if the medication is contributing to the sleep issues and how to address the problem if it is a factor.

Exercise

The research is clear – one of the most important things anyone with ADHD can do to naturally manage their symptoms is to make exercise a regular part of their life. Study after study shows improvements in concentration, attention, academic performance, distractibility, focus, hyperactivity, and overall behavior management when children and adults with ADHD engage in regular physical exercise.

The reason exercise is so beneficial to those with ADHD is that it helps activate the executive functions in the brain. It also helps teach the skills many with ADHD need to overcome the challenges they face so that they can be successful. Skills like resilience, persistence, and continuing on after failing are all things that can be learned in physically demanding activities like sports, exercise programs, and active hobbies.

Additionally, exercise boosts self-confidence. Studies with rats have shown that simply exercising makes experiencing feelings of hopelessness less likely. These are both important factors for people with ADHD who are very likely to struggle with depression and anxiety resulting from the difficulties they experience because of the disorder.

The key to the benefits those with ADHD get from exercising stems from our biology. When we participate in active pursuits like walking or running, chemicals are released by the brain. Dopamine, the chemical that people with ADHD generally do not have enough of to begin with, is one of those chemicals. Exercise also creates endorphins which help regulate and elevate mood. Flooding the brain with endorphins and elevating dopamine levels increases focus, makes it easier to pay attention, and improves alertness.

People with ADHD don't need to be exercise fanatics in order to get the benefit of regular exercise. Experts agree that 30 minutes of sustained activity at least four times a week is enough to provide these benefits.

The best way to incorporate this kind of exercise is to choose an active pursuit that is fun and enjoyable. The goal is to get the exercise, which doesn't mean the person with ADHD has to run or work out at a gym. It is important to find something that is interesting enough that they will want to participate. Playing team sports like soccer, baseball, softball, and basketball, even for adults, can be a great way to get in the right amount of exercise in a way that is fun and exciting. This kind of exercise can also help boost confidence and teach social skills for those with the disorder who struggle in those areas.

However, some people with ADHD are wary of team sports where social interaction is required or the success of the team rests on the performance of the individual. If these things are a concern, choose something that doesn't create these kinds of anxiety. While these are skills that most with ADHD could benefit from improving, if social or performance anxiety makes participation unpleasant, it is better to seek other ways to boost those skills so that they get the benefit of the exercise.

The best kinds of activities for people with ADHD are those that require sustain focus and mind-body connection. These are things like karate, ballet, gymnastics, swimming, rock climbing, yoga, tai chi, and dancing. Studies have shown that these types of activities give the executive functions responsible for focus and attention a good workout, which strengthens them for use in other areas.

Additionally, research has shown that when people with ADHD participate in yoga or tai chi, they experience improvements with hyperactivity, emotional regulation, and anxiety.

As an added benefit, regular exercise also helps reduce and manage stress and promotes sleep.

Therapy

Many people with ADHD struggle with emotional disregulation, low self-esteem, communication, social interactions, and other mental health disorders. Where coaching can help those with ADHD implement new habits and take action to make positive behavior modifications, therapy can help those with the disorder understand and manage the emotional side of their symptoms.

Cognitive behavioral therapy, play therapy, and psychotherapy can all help those with ADHD understand the role their emotions play in their symptoms. These treatment options can help those that struggle with emotional disregulation learn to identify, manage, and deal with their emotions more appropriately.

For those people with ADHD who struggle socially, this kind of treatment provides the opportunity to learn the social skills they are lacking and to practice those skills in a supportive environment. A therapy group filled with peers can be an effective way for those with ADHD to develop their social skills among people who understand them. By providing a safe space to practice things like having a conversation or resolving a conflict, this kind of treatment setting can make it possible for those with ADHD to gain the skills they need to be more successful in the outside world.

Therapy, both in an individual and group setting, can also help overcome self-esteem issues which can be a critical step for those with ADHD. One of the things that happens when someone with ADHD has low self-esteem is that they are less willing to try new things that might help them better manage their symptoms. This unwillingness comes from their fear of failing and can make it impossible for them to make meaningful progress in creating the kind of life they want. Additionally, low self-esteem makes people with ADHD more vulnerable to negative influences which can be dangerous for a group where the rate of substance abuse is already higher than average.

For those with other mental health conditions like anxiety, depression, or OCD, therapy helps ensure that all mental health conditions are being treated together. Research has shown that treating one mental health condition in people where more than one condition is present is ineffective. This is especially true for those struggling with substance abuse in addition to their ADHD. Because many of the mental health conditions that are frequently co-morbid with ADHD may result from the symptoms of the underlying ADHD, they must be treated together in a cohesive manner in order for the treatment to be effective. In these cases, working with a mental health professional is imperative in order to achieve results, regardless of whether or not any of the conditions are being treated by medication.

One of the most important things anyone with ADHD can achieve by including therapy in their management plan is new coping strategies for handling challenging situations. Unfortunately, many people with ADHD develop unhealthy ways of coping with the stress and emotional turmoil they experience because of the disorder. This is why the rate of substance abuse is so much higher for those with ADHD than it is for the general population. Replacing unhealthy coping mechanisms with positive, healthy coping strategies can make a significant difference in all areas of that person's life.

Another type of therapy that can be very beneficial for those with ADHD and their families is participation in a support group. People with ADHD often feel alone and isolated because the people around them don't understand what it is like to have ADHD. Joining a support group surrounds that person with other people who can provide the support and understanding that people who do not have ADHD cannot provide. Sharing experiences, frustrations, and successes with others who are dealing with the same challenges develops a sense of camaraderie that helps alleviates feelings of loneliness and isolation.

Diet

While there is no scientific evidence that specific foods cause ADHD, this doesn't mean that diet doesn't play a part in the symptoms someone with the condition experiences. Diet does play a role in symptom severity for the same reason that sleep can impact symptoms – stress on the body.

In the chapter on stress management, the relationship between stress and ADHD symptoms was explained, including the fact that anything that stresses the body can make symptoms worse. Diet can put a lot of stress on the body. Good nutrition is important for everyone. When people don't eat a healthy diet, their body doesn't have the nutrition it needs to operate optimally. Eating too much or eating the wrong things can increase the severity of ADHD symptoms because of the stress it causes on the body.

Food Sensitivities

In addition to eating a healthy, balanced diet, people with ADHD need to pay particular attention to food sensitivities as these often hidden conditions can cause tremendous stress on the system and exacerbate symptoms. The first step in using diet as a way to manage symptoms is to understand which foods cause symptoms to be worse and which seem to make them better. There are two ways to figure this out.

The first is to use the kind of test used to determine if a person has any common food allergies. It's called The Elimination Diet and Challenge Test. To determine if there is a sensitivity or allergy to any of the most common allergenic foods, they are all eliminated from the diet for a period of time and then added back in one at a time. The most common food sensitivities/allergies are milk, eggs, nuts, wheat, citric acid, and soy. In addition, people with ADHD may consider including refined sugar and caffeine in their elimination test as sensitivities to these foods can also make symptoms worse.

During the elimination part of the test, it is important to keep track of all food and drink and to track ADHD symptoms. Most people continue with the elimination diet for two or three weeks. Over that time, if ADHD symptoms seem to improve, there may be food sensitivity at play. If there isn't any improvement, it is unlikely that food sensitivity is affecting symptoms, and people may choose to go back to their regular eating habits without completing the second half of the test.

After two or three weeks, each eliminated food is added back into the diet, one at a time with three to five days elapsing before the next food is added. Keeping track of ADHD symptoms during this time will help highlight any areas where a specific food seems to make symptoms worse or better. Once all the foods have been added back in, reviewing results may indicate that permanently eliminating one or more of the foods being tested will provide symptom relief.

The second way to test for food allergies is to do the same type of elimination testing, but this time do it by eliminating only one food at a time. For example, eliminating sugar from the diet for two weeks then adding it back in for a week before moving on to the next potential allergen. Tracking food and beverages and ADHD symptoms is just as important for this kind of testing.

Brain Food

In addition to eating a balanced diet and looking for food sensitivities, people with ADHD can use food to boost their brain power by eating more "brain food." Protein-rich foods like lean meat, nuts, soy, and dairy products provide the raw materials needed to make the neurotransmitters the brain uses for cell to cell communication. High protein diets also help prevent blood sugar spikes that can exacerbate problems with hyperactivity, especially in those who are sensitive to sugar.

Reducing the amount of sugar in the diet, regardless of any existing sensitivities, is also important because too much sugar puts a lot of stress on the body. Blood sugar spikes and drops cause mood swings in anyone and for those with ADHD who already struggle with emotional disregulation, these spikes and cause erratic behavior and damaging outbursts.

Although the science isn't yet there to support it, there is a strong belief that some preservative and artificial colorings can also exacerbate ADHD symptoms. Foods that contain the following artificial ingredients may increase hyperactivity in some people.

- Sodium benzoate
- FD&C Yellow No. 6
- D&C Yellow No. 10
- FD&C Yellow No. 5
- FD&C Red No. 40

If sensitivity is suspected, using the elimination diet and challenge test can help pinpoint which ingredients, if any, increase hyperactivity or other symptoms.

Supplements and Herbs

Many people with ADHD look to supplements to help with symptom management, even though the science and research haven't yet established whether or not the perceived or attributed benefits actually exist. For this reason, it is important to discuss the use of any vitamin or supplement with a medical doctor before adding it to an ADHD management program. Here are the most commonly used supplements for ADHD symptom support and management.

Fish Oil

Research suggests that not having enough omega-3 fatty acids in the diet can exacerbate some ADHD symptoms. These fats, which are found in things like fish and tree nuts, are important to brain function. Studies so far suggest that some people with ADHD may see symptom improvement when they increase their dietary intake of omega-3s or use fish oil supplements that are high in omega-3s.

B Vitamins

Research has shown that when children have low levels of the B vitamins in their blood, increasing those levels with supplements causes a jump in IQ and a decrease in both aggressive and anti-social behavior. This result is believed to result from an increase in dopamine caused by one or more of the B vitamins.

Zinc

Research has shown that low levels of zinc can cause or increase problems with attention. This mineral is also important in the production of dopamine in the brain and not having enough zinc could impede dopamine production.

Iron

Iron is another mineral that is important for the production of dopamine. One study found more than 80% of children with ADHD had low ferritin levels (a measurement of iron level) which is significantly higher than the incidence seen in those without ADHD. Not having enough iron has been shown to cause other cognitive deficits in other studies.

Picamilon

This supplement uses niacin (one of the B vitamins) and other ingredients to improve blood flow to the brain. It also produces a mild stimulating effect which can help increase both alertness and attention in those with ADHD.

Gingko and Ginseng

Gingko can help with memory challenges and is believed to improve mental sharpness. Ginseng is said to support the production of dopamine in the brain. When used together, some benefit to those with ADHD has been documented.

Melatonin

Melatonin is a hormone produced in the body that helps to control the sleep and wake cycles of humans. The release of melatonin is triggered by light exposure, levels rise at night as the sun goes down, which tells the body it is time to go to sleep. When the sun comes up and light exposure increases, melatonin levels drop, which signifies that it is time to wake up. Melatonin supplements can be beneficial in helping those with ADHD who struggle with sleep.

Conclusion

Thank you again for purchasing this book!

I hope it was valuable to you in explaining the natural and holistic treatment options for ADHD.

With the information provided in this guide, you have the tools to tackle some of the most damaging symptoms of ADHD, even if you choose not to use pharmaceuticals. Using these alternative treatments, you can create an ADHD management program tailored to your individual needs. Remember, understanding and knowledge are the best medicine!

Finally, if you enjoyed this book, please take the time to share your thoughts and post a review on Amazon. It'd be greatly appreciated!

Thank you and good luck!

Christine Weil

Check out some of Christine's other books!!!

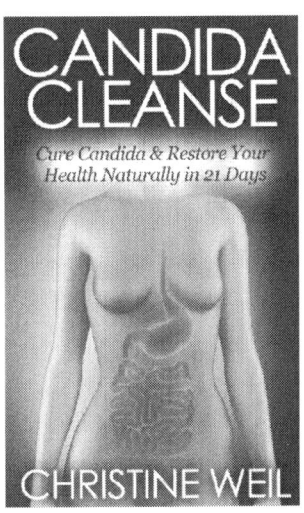

http://www.amazon.com/dp/B00IIRQH9K

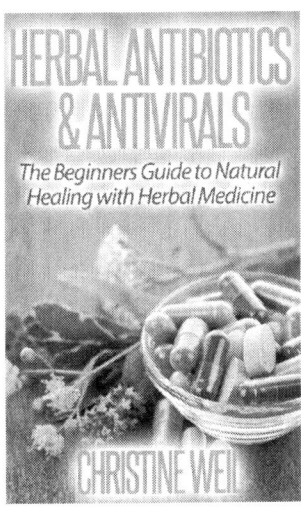

http://www.amazon.com/dp/B00J2F1QDO

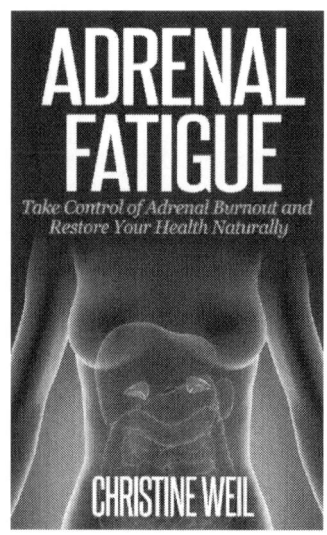

http://www.amazon.com/dp/B00J8SHS6E

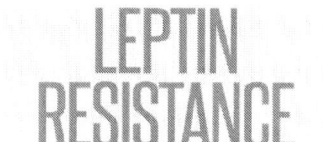

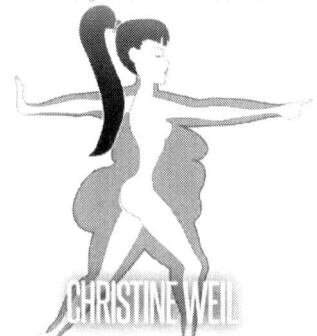

http://www.amazon.com/dp/B00J8UNBWW

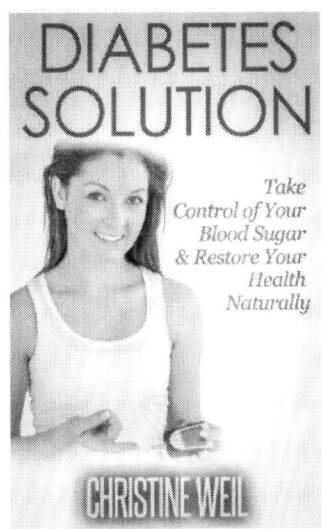

http://www.amazon.com/dp/B00KCAAKOO

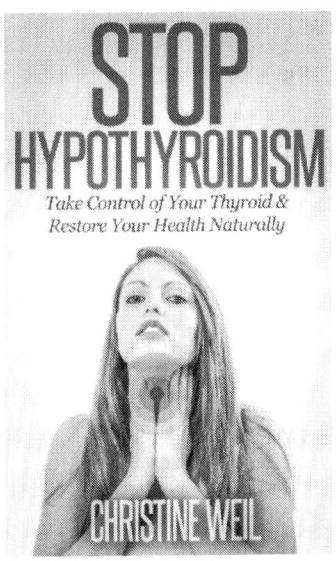

http://www.amazon.com/dp/B00KGI6TEC

34365726R00020

Printed in Great Britain
by Amazon